RELAXATION AND E:
FOR CHILDBIRTH

GW00361007

RELAXATION AND EXERCISE FOR CHILDBIRTH

The Late **HELEN HEARDMAN**
Diploma Bedford Physical Training College;
Chartered Physiotherapist (Teacher's certificate)

Revised and re-edited by

MARIA EBNER M.C.S.P., Dip.T.P.
Diploma in Physical Education (Vienna
University). Former Principal of the School and
Department of Physiotherapy of the United Leeds
Hospitals

Foreword by

JOSEPHINE BARNES
D.B.E., M.A., D.M., F.R.C.P., F.R.C.S.,
F.R.C.O.G. (Hon), F.R.C.P. (Ireland) President,
Association of Chartered Physiotherapists in
Obstetrics and Gynaecology

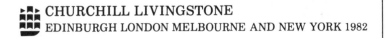 **CHURCHILL LIVINGSTONE**
EDINBURGH LONDON MELBOURNE AND NEW YORK 1982

CHURCHILL LIVINGSTONE
Medical Division of Longman Group UK Limited

Distributed in the United States of America by Churchill
Livingstone Inc., 19 West 44th Street, New York, N.Y.
10036, and by associated companies, branches
and representatives throughout the world.

First Edition 1950
Second Edition 1959
Third Edition 1966
Fourth Edition 1974
Fifth Edition revised by Maria Ebner 1982
Reprinted 1986

ISBN 0-443-02194-5

British Library Cataloguing in Publication Data
Heardman, Helen
  Relaxation and exercise for childbirth—5th ed.—
  (Churchill Livingstone patient handbook)
  1. Childbirth—Psychology—Handbook, manuals, etc.
  I. Title II. Ebner, Maria
  618.2′4   RG661

Library of Congress Catalog Card Number 81-68600

Produced by Longman Singapore Publishers Pte Ltd
Printed in Singapore

FOREWORD

This is the fifth edition of a well known and successful booklet the purpose of which is to help women and their husbands to prepare for the act of childbirth.

The work of the obstetrician Grantley Dick Read which began in the 1930s first introduced the idea that women should prepare mentally and physically for the act of childbirth and that this preparation, combined with the practice of relaxation, could do much to make childbirth a rewarding experience and one to be looked forward to, a great change from the fear and dread felt by so many in the past.

Grantley Dick Read's ideas were taken up by his disciple Helen Heardman, a physiotherapist who made childbirth preparation her life's work and eventually died tragically in a road accident on her way to the labour of one of her patients. This booklet is her lasting memorial and it has been skilfully revised by Maria Ebner.

The booklet recognises the fact that now the great majority of births take place in hospital. Most births are still normal but the woman entering a maternity hospital may have to face many new developments in maternity care. Up to 10 percent of babies are now born by Caesarean section and forceps delivery is used freely in cases of difficulty or of danger to the unborn baby. There is a wide range of measures for the relief of pain in labour where necessary, including drugs such as pethidine or epidural analgesia which can render childbirth virtually pain-free. Episiotomy, an incision to expedite delivery is widely used. Induction of labour is now being used less frequently but still may be necessary in some situations. It is now usual for the mother to receive a drip, by which fluid is 'dripped' into a vein to prevent dehydration and acidosis. Pitocin may be added to expedite delivery. The study of the condition of the unborn baby by fetal monitoring is also widely used. The mother must understand that these techniques are undertaken in the interest of mother and baby. It is important that due explanation of their use is given by the staff. It must be emphasised that as a result of developments in maternity care childbirth is now safer for mother and baby than ever before. These new techniques do not conflict with the idea that every mother should prepare for normal childbirth which will be achieved in the majority and intervention will only take place when the life or safety of either mother or baby is threatened.

Most maternity clinics now provide classes for training in childbirth. These should include parenthood classes for mothers and fathers and techniques used in the labour ward should be clearly and thoroughly explained. This booklet is designed to supplement instruction given by physiotherapists, midwives and doctors. It is also intended for use by those mothers who for one reason or another are unable to attend classes.

It concentrates on the basic needs of childbirth preparation, breathing, relaxation, posture and exercises; it also gives a clear and simple account of normal labour and the part to be played by the mother. The well-prepared woman can hope, not only to give birth more easily, but to recover from the effects of childbirth, whether normal or abnormal, more rapidly and thus be fit to care for her baby and the rest of her family.

Over the years many women and their husbands, who can play a part in helping their wives, have found this booklet invaluable and this new and improved edition is warmly welcomed.

London, 1982   *Josephine Barnes*

PREFACE

Childbearing — pregnancy, labour and the puerperium — is a natural event in a woman's life and it should be possible for her to pass through its stages without injury to her health. Doctors, midwives, health visitors and physiotherapists make a positive contribution to this end.

A new edition of this booklet provides the opportunity to adapt it to changed economic and social conditions, and changed attitudes to natural childbirth. I am grateful to the publishers to be given this opportunity.

Leeds, 1982   *Maria Ebner*

CONTENTS

1. INTRODUCTION

Since the previous revision of this booklet a number of economic and social aspects of life have fundamentally changed. The majority of pregnant women are now delivered in hospital maternity units or in general practitioner's units. The hospital stay is in many cases very short, often only 48 hours, and the mother returns home to receive the necessary immediate aftercare from the community midwife. Her further welfare is then entrusted to the health visitor and G.P. Naturally, these changes have necessitated very close co-operation between involved parties to avoid conflicting or confusing instruction.

It is common for expectant women to stay at work very much longer and it is therefore very important that, early in her pregnancy, an expectant mother has at her disposal information about diet, basic breathing, and posture at work and at leisure. Later in her pregnancy she will be able to attend regular classes. This booklet aims to cater particularly for the mother in this situation so that damage to her health may be avoided and that good dietary habits are established to create favourable conditions for the baby's development.

During the past years many more classes have been made available in hospitals and community centres and I hope we are approaching the day when every pregnant woman will have the opportunity of receiving the necessary help to make pregnancy, labour and the puerperium (the first few weeks after childbirth) a happy time. The increase in the number of fathers who are taking a more active part in providing favourable conditions for the arrival and development of the child is also a good sign.

After these preliminary remarks may I address myself directly to mothers and fathers? If your baby is to be born naturally, each of the following factors is of great importance:

1. Good health, in the father as well as in the mother. When the parents are healthy, conditions remain normal 95 per cent of the time.
2. Early booking of a doctor and midwife, or a place in a hospital in which you can place your confidence and whose instructions you will follow implicitly. It is well to have a clear understanding about your desire to have a natural childbirth and the willingness of the attendants to help you to achieve it.
3. A fearless acceptance of the months of pregnancy as a period of training and preparation for all that will follow.

It is also important to learn what to expect — how babies are conceived, how they develop and how they are born; how the mother's body adapts to the presence of the developing baby; and what both parents can do to promote the health of the baby. All this can be learned from the doctor, midwife, health visitor and physiotherapist at classes.

This booklet is intended to supplement and be a reminder of these classes; it should also be a considerable help where classes are not available. Daily practice of relaxation and exercises outlined in this booklet is essential so the mother can prepare her body for labour and learn to breathe and relax at the proper times during labour in order to help the natural progress of childbirth. This physical training promotes good health, poise, good posture and good body mechanics during and after pregnancy. It should not, however, be attempted without the consent of the doctor who knows about the mother's physical condition.

How to use this book?

You and your husband may find yourself reading these words at any stage of your pregnancy; if it is towards the beginning you will have plenty of time to digest and practice the exercises, especially if an early class can be arranged in your area. The nearer to the expected date it is, the less time you will have and it may be wise to concentrate on breathing, relaxation and muscle control. Learn one exercise properly per day; then repeat it daily and finally build this up to three times daily. If possible try to repeat the whole series twice a day. Many of the exercises can be fitted in while doing other things.

Content of the early class

1. Diet. More detailed information may be given by the doctor, the midwife or the health visitor. Sensible diet throughout pregnancy is very important as overeating must be avoided; it should contain plenty of protein, i.e. meat, fish, cheese, eggs and milk and adequate amounts of fresh fruits and vegetables including salads; starchy foods such as bread, potatoes, cakes and sweets should be eaten in moderation as these are primarily responsible for excessive weight gain.
2. Abdominal breathing (see exercise 1 (a), page 5).
3. Foot exercises whenever sitting down (see exercise 2, page 7).
4. Relaxation in side-lying before sleep (see exercise 3, page 8).
5. Pelvic tilting in sitting (see exercise 8, page 18).
6. Posture whenever you are standing (see exercise 9, page 20).

2. RELAXATION AND EXERCISE FOR NATURAL CHILDBIRTH

This text will be easier to understand if you study the diagrams of the baby in the mother's body and the relative position of the organs in her pelvis (see Figs. 1 and 2).

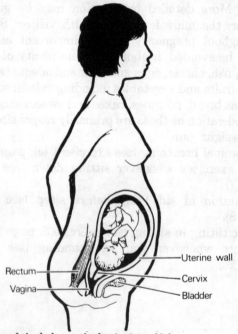

Rectum

Vagina

Uterine wall

Cervix

Bladder

Fig. 1 Position of the baby at the beginning of labour.

The exercises are listed in the order of their importance, and each should be tried out and made perfect before proceeding to the next. The bladder should be emptied before starting any exercises.

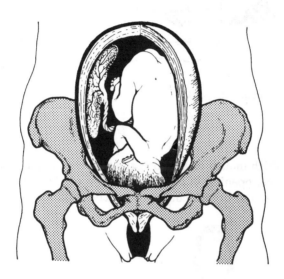

Fig. 2 Baby ready to pass through the pelvis when labour begins.

Exercise 1: breathing

Lie (on a rug on the floor, or on a bed which does not sag) on the back with knees bent, and feet flat on the floor or bed, one or two pillows under the head. These exercises can also be done on a chair or in the bath.

(a) With mouth closed, breathe gently in and out, keeping quite loose and letting the abdominal wall rise up with the

5

indrawn breath and drop down with the outgoing one. This must be practised every day. (Fig. 3).

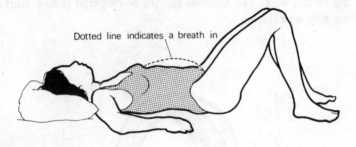

Dotted line indicates a breath in

Fig. 3 Breathing (a).

(b) With mouth closed, breathe slowly to expand the ribs sideways, opening out the inverted V of the ribs in front. Again let the breath come out gently. (Fig. 4)

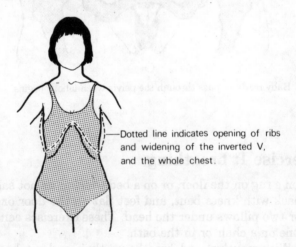

Dotted line indicates opening of ribs and widening of the inverted V, and the whole chest.

Fig. 4 Breathing (b).

6

(c) With mouth slightly open, breathe in more quickly, lifting up the sternum or breastbone and letting it lower again. This type of breathing is shallower and therefore quicker and therefore necessitates breathing through the nose and mouth together to get more air in during a shorter period of time. This breathing is not a normal breathing but is learned for use during the later part of labour. (Fig. 5.)

These breathing exercises can be done in the bath, or in bed before getting up or going to sleep at night; in the latter case (c) should be left out.

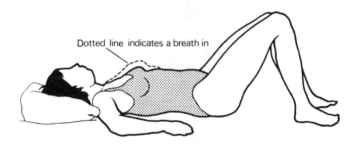

Dotted line indicates a breath in

Fig. 5 Breathing (c).

Exercise 2: foot exercises

The growing baby and the increasing bodyweight very often cause pain and circulatory difficulties in the feet and legs. Simple foot exercises can help to prevent this.

Sitting on a chair with feet supported on a stool or lying.
(a) Bend and stretch ankles.
(b) Bend and stretch toes.
(c) Roll feet round in circles in both directions.
These exercises should be done as often as possible.

7

Exercise 3: relaxation

Lie on the floor on one side, head on pillow, not shoulders, eyes and mouth gently closed, back and neck well bowed forward, under arm behind the back and bent at the elbow and wrist, top arm also bent lying on the floor (or pillow) in front, top leg should be bent at hip, knee and ankle and placed in front of the bottom leg which is bent in the same manner. (Fig. 6).

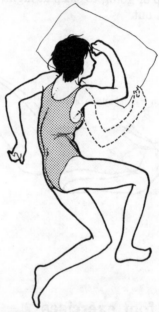

Fig. 6 Relaxation.

This is usually found to be the most comfortable and effective position for relaxing during pregnancy, because all parts of the body rest on a firm support, so no muscle is tense because it has to work to carry the weight of any part of the body. All joints are loosely bent, so no muscle is unwittingly drawn taut across a joint. (If difficulty is found with the position, put further cushions under any uncomfortable part, but practise on a firm surface.)

8

(*a*) Contract and relax each group of muscles in turn, as follows:

Left leg—Squeeze down the toes—relax.
  Bend down the ankle—relax.
  Bend up the ankle—relax.
  Straighten the knee a little way—relax.
  Bend the knee a little way—relax.
  Tighten the hip muscle that you sit on—relax.

Right leg—Do the same as with the left leg.

Left arm—Stretch the fingers—relax.
  Bend elbow a little way—relax.
  Straighten elbow a little way—relax.
  Tighten the shoulder muscle on which you are lying—relax.

Right arm—Do the same as with the left arm.

Face—Let all the muscles of face and neck (eyes, mouth, nose, forehead) sag.

(*b*) When the whole body feels loose and sagging begin to breathe consciously, naturally and quietly (listening inwardly to what you are doing).

(*c*) As you breathe, say to yourself, 'in—out', making each word last the appropriate movement of breath. The rhythm of the breathing releases mental tensions and keeping your mind on the 'in—out' prevents any worrisome or disturbing thoughts from creeping in to destroy the peace of mind which is essential for complete relaxation.

When the relaxation is good the body begins to feel very comfortable, the floor seems soft and you seem to be as light as a feather—finally a feeling as of the floor rising up under the body like a lift is experienced. Sleep may, and if the time is right usually will, follow such relaxation.

During relaxation the circulation is at its slowest. The heart, therefore, must be brought back gradually to its regular work, so small muscle movements like clenching hands and feet must be done, followed by stretching of legs and arms and a gradual sitting up before standing after this exercise. If you do not do this, you may feel faint or giddy.

As soon as you learn to relax completely, muscle group by muscle group, try relaxing all over at once, as you will want to be able, during the first stage of labour, to relax completely the moment a contraction begins. This controlled relaxation is nature's desire for the first stage of labour and must be used each time the uterus contracts. Only thus can the uterine muscle fibres act freely to open the cervix without pain. (See Chapter 3.)

The best time to practise relaxation is daily after the midday meal, at the beginning of an afternoon rest and at night when getting ready to go to sleep. Remember always the three principles of relaxation:

1. Full support for all parts of the body.
2. No muscle tension anywhere—joints, face, hands, feet, etc.
3. Peace of mind.

Once you feel you have acquired some degree of relaxation, try a short period of the breathing described in Exercise 1 (a), since this is the method you will use in the first stage of labour when lying in the relaxation position.

Exercise 4: alternative relaxation positions

A. Lying on the back with a pillow under the head, two pillows under the knees, a pillow supporting the feet, the arms bent at the elbows and resting on the pillows. (The head pillow should prevent the head from rolling to either side.) (Fig. 7.)

Apply the three principles of Exercise 3 and relax. Use it sometimes instead of lying on the side at the relaxation period.

10

B. In an armchair with feet on the floor or a footstool, a pillow under the head, thighs fully supported, forearms supported along the arms of the chair. (Fig. 8.)

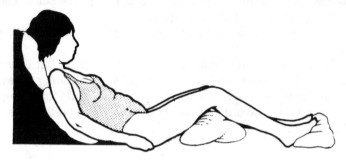

Fig. 7 Relaxation. Alternative position.

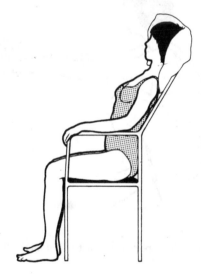

Fig. 8 Relaxation. Alternative position.

Apply the three principles of Exercise 3 and relax.

Practise relaxing in these positions because it may not always be possible to lie on the side as in Exercise 3 when in labour.

Exercise 5: squatting

Standing with the feet flat on the floor parallel and about 18 inches apart holding on to a firm support (e.g. the sink). The firm support is very important.

Squat right back on to the heels, starting with outward rotation of the knees.

At first the balance may be difficult to acquire, but every day it will be easier, and some small jobs like cleaning shoes, peeling potatoes, tidying a draw, can be done while squatting. If it is found to be difficult, wear shoes with flat heels at first. (Figs. 9–11).

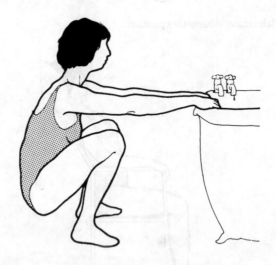

Fig. 9 Squatting with support. Feet must be flat on the floor and 18 inches apart.

This is the position which keeps the back supple which is essential for labour. It is assumed by primitive women during childbirth. Getting accustomed to this position during pregnancy by regular and repeated squatting keeps the back

12

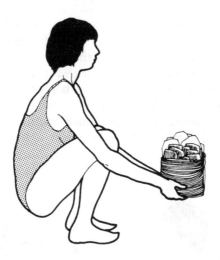

Fig. 10 Squatting to lift an object.

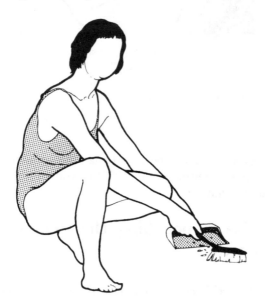

Fig. 11 Low-level housework.

13

supple, prevents future backache and may help to relieve constipation which is often a problem during pregnancy. The position is now modified for labour for the comfort of the mother. She is now lying down with the knees bent, the back well supported from behind by a back support and pillow. The ideal position is when the husband is present during labour to support the woman under both shoulders, giving her physical comfort and the comfort of his presence. (Fig. 12.)

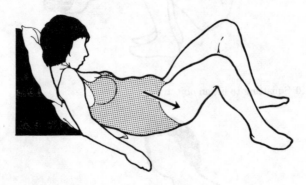

Fig. 12 Squatting applied to delivery.

However, it should be noted that the squatting position should be attempted gradually if the woman is not used to it before pregnancy.

Exercise 6: polishing the floor on hands and knees

On hands and knees (see exercise 8B for correct position).

Move round the room dusting or polishing the floor.

14

The abdominal organs are all attached to the backbone by strong membranes. In this position these organs hang from the backbone like clothes on a line, instead of hanging, as they do when you are upright, like a flag on a pole. When they are like a flag on a pole they tend to fall down towards the pelvis and press on the great blood vessels and nerves. This hands and knees position relieves that pressure. Moving around in this position limbers and loosens the joints of spine and hips and strengthens the abdominal muscles which is desirable in pregnancy as well as in labour.

Exercise 7: contraction and relaxation of the pelvic floor muscles

Lie on the back with knees and feet flat on the floor.

(a) Squeeze the two buttock muscles together and draw the exit of the back-passage in as if to prevent a bowel action. Count six slowly and slowly relax. Do this until the action is strong and perfect.

(b) While doing (a) pull up as though preventing a bladder action and again count six slowly and then slowly relax both contractions.

(c) Tighten the muscles around the bladder and vaginal passage only, as though preventing a bladder action, counting six slowly again and slowly relax.

The pelvis, through which the baby must pass as it is being born, has a muscular floor with three openings — the urethra, the vaginal outlet, and the anus. These pelvic floor muscles must be elastic for natural childbirth, so that when relaxed they will stretch to let the child pass through comfortably and will then contract to support the pelvic organs after the baby is born. Muscle is living elastic and unlike the commercial kind becomes more elastic with careful and repeated contraction and relaxation.

Exercise (c) particularly increases this elasticity and prepares the mother to relax these muscles during labour and should therefore be done daily and often. It can be practised

15

quite easily standing with heels and toes together while washing dishes, waiting in a queue etc., also while sitting.

Exercise 8: pelvic tilting

Pelvic tilting can be done in many positions. The three described are the simplest and most useful during pregnancy.

A. Lie on the back with knees bent, and feet flat on bed or floor, head supported on one or two pillows.

(*a*) Tighten the buttock muscles and simultaneously draw in the lower abdominal wall, pressing the back firmly on to the floor. (Fig. 13.)

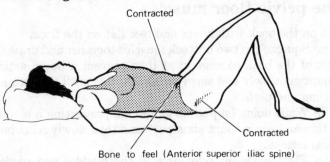

Contracted

Contracted

Bone to feel (Anterior superior iliac spine)

Fig. 13 Tilting up.

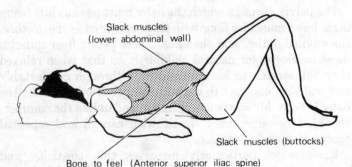

Slack muscles (lower abdominal wall)

Slack muscles (buttocks)

Bone to feel (Anterior superior iliac spine)

Fig. 14 Tilting down.

16

(*b*) Relax both groups of muscles gently and contract the lower back muscles to make a tunnel under them. (Fig. 14.)

(*c*) After attempting this several times find the bones above either hip in front and test whether these go down towards the feet with the hollow back and come up towards the head with the flat one. If so, the pelvis is tilting correctly.

Warning: Breathe in and out all the time naturally and keep the shoulders and hips firmly on the floor.

This exercise has to be done specially as there is no everyday movement to correspond. A good time to practise it is before the relaxation period.

Then try this second position:

B. On the hands and knees with hands directly below the shoulders and the knees directly below the hips, keeping all angles true right angles. (Fig. 15.)

Tilt the pelvis by contracting buttock muscles and the low abdominal muscles, so that the back assumes a humped-up appearance like a cat spitting (Fig. 16), then relax both groups so that the back become straight again. (Fig. 15).

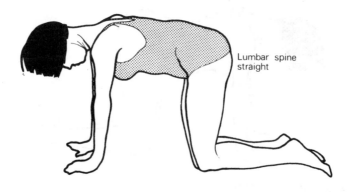

Lumbar spine straight

Fig. 15 Starting position for pelvic tilting in prone kneeling.

Warning: This exercise should not be carried to the point where the spine becomes hollowed. (Fig. 17.)

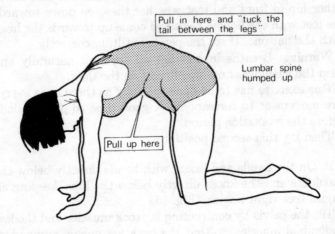

Pull in here and "tuck the tail between the legs"

Lumbar spine humped up

Pull up here

Fig. 16 Tilting up.

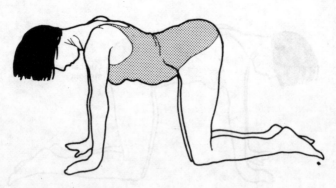

Fig. 17 Incorrect position.

C. Sitting forward on a stool or chair with hands grasping the back of the stool or chair. (Fig. 18.)

18

It is essential to sit forward on the stool to allow some of the weight to be taken on the feet. The position of the hands fixes the thoracic spine (upper part of the spine) and therefore isolates the movement to the lumbar region (lower part of the spine).

Contract the buttock and abdominal muscles to tilt the pelvis backwards, contract the back and hip muscles to tilt the pelvis in the opposite direction—return to the starting position.

This type of pelvic tilting can easily be fitted in during the day whenever you sit down.

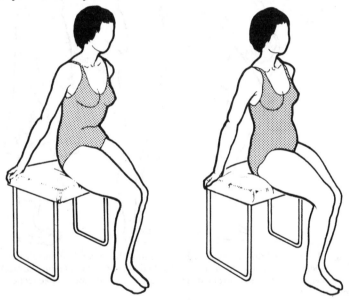

Fig. 18 Pelvic tilting in sitting position.

This pelvic tilting has value for improving posture and strengthening the abdominal muscles. It is also of value in pregnancy because bad posture is closely connected with the preventable backache which is frequently worrying to expectant mothers. It is extremely rare in women who can and do control the pelvis and posture.

19

Exercise 9: posture correction

When the pelvic tilting is appreciated in the other positions, try it standing.

Stand firmly with feet nearly parallel and all toes pressed against the floor, with weight well over the arches of the feet.

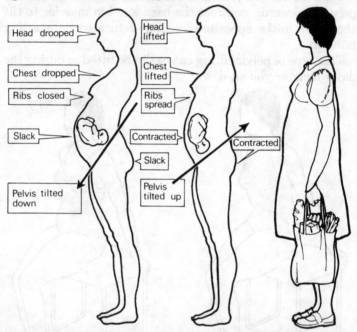

Head drooped

Chest dropped

Ribs closed

Slack

Pelvis tilted down

Head lifted

Chest lifted

Ribs spread

Contracted

Slack

Pelvis tilted up

Contracted

Fig. 19 The tilted-down pelvis with baby using the abdominal muscles as a hammock and causing them to be stretched. The weight falls on the back muscles which become strained and lead to the well-known backache of pregnancy.

Fig 20 The abdominal muscles holding the baby in the tilted-up pelvis. A perfect balance of muscle back and front.

Tilt the pelvis upward. Open out the chest by rib-spread breathing as in Exercise 1 (b) and see that the breasts are carried well forward over the abdomen. Then lift the head towards the roof as if it were suspended from above. (Fig. 20.)

20

Breathe easily, conquering the tendency to hold the breath which often comes during muscular effort.

A woman carrying her child should radiate good health and happiness and have a noticeable grace of movement and poise of body at all times. Good posture brings big dividends in health and appearance during and after pregnancy. The correct position of the pelvis is the foundation of good posture.

Exercise 10: breathing

During labour the mother's part in physical terms, consists very largely in a control of breathing. Try the following variations of Exercise 1.

(*d*) Lying on the back with knees bent and feet flat, head and shoulders supported by pillows. Practising changing from Breathing 1 (*a*) to Breathing 1 (*c*) i.e. Take a deep breath in letting the abdominal wall rise and immediately release the air then continue to breathe as in 1 (*c*) with open mouth letting the breast bone rise and lower again.

(*e*) Same position—mouth open. Draw one quick deep breath, then close the mouth and hold the breath, counting ten slowly. At the end of this period let the breath go quickly and naturally. Repeat holding the breath gradually for longer periods up to 25 counts.

(*f*) Same position as above. Draw and release a number of quick and shallow breaths. This creates a panting effect, with continuously vibrating abdomen.

(*g*) Breathing for expulsion. All expulsive acts take place using the same 'pattern'. The upward expulsive acts are sneezing, coughing, vomitting, the downward ones are defaecation (emptying the bowels), micturition (emptying the bladder), parturition (emptying the uterus). The uterus can only be emptied when the cervix is open at the end of the first stage of labour (see Chapter 3) but the method is similar to emptying the bowels. Therefore every time you empty your bowels draw a breath as described under (e), then hold it and finally bear down and use the expulsive act. It will be easier with 2 footstools about 12 inches high placed in front of the lavatory seat on which to place your feet. You are then in a position similar to squatting, which is recognised as the position in which the downward expulsive acts occur with greatest thoroughness and ease.

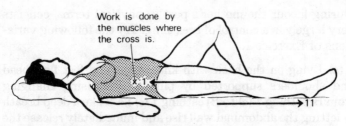

Work is done by the muscles where the cross is.

The straight leg is drawn along the floor in the direction of arrow 1, and then pushed down in the direction of arrow 11. The movement in the spine can be increased by moving the head and shoulders towards the right leg, reaching down it with the right arm.

Fig. 21 Working waist muscles.

Exercise 11: pelvic tilting sideways and rotation

A. Pelvic tilting sideways. Lie on the back with one leg bent and the other straight, arms spread sideways, palms on the floor, tilting the pelvis up by making the waist line firm and much more curved inwards. Then let the leg return to its previous position. (Fig. 21.)

Once the muscle action has been learned, this exercise can be done standing. Care must be taken to see that the straight leg is truly drawn up to make the waist line curve in.

B. Pelvic rotation. Lie on the back as in exercise 11A. Roll the bent knee over the straight leg in an attempt to touch the floor with it; on returning relax the bent leg slowly so that the knee touches the floor on the same side. During the second part of this exercise, the muscles on the inside of the thigh and the pelvic floor muscles should be completely relaxed. (Fig. 22.)

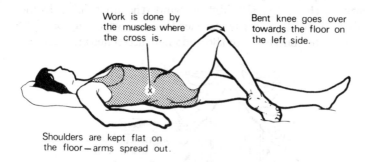

Work is done by the muscles where the cross is.

Bent knee goes over towards the floor on the left side.

Shoulders are kept flat on the floor—arms spread out.

Fig. 22 Working oblique abdominal muscles.

Warning: The abdomen must be drawn in before beginning both exercises or the wrong set of muscles will be used.

The different slants of the different layers of the abdominal muscles (as shown in the sketches) allow them to move the trunk in different directions—bend it forwards, or sideways and turn it—and to move the pelvis—tilt it upward, tilt it sideways or rotate it. This bending, turning, tilting and rotating strengthens the abdominal muscles that stretch as the baby grows and must be kept strong and elastic to hold the enlarging uterus in good position. They are used also during the expulsive efforts of the second stage of labour. When these abdominal muscles are used simultaneously and the chest and pelvis kept still they draw in the abdominal wall at the sides and front and are therefore often referred to in this connection as 'nature's corset'. Nature, it will be seen, has provided the best type of corset—a 'three-way stretch'.

Practise these exercises regularly to keep those abdominal muscles in good trim and so avoid the necessity for a maternity corset. (If, however, the weight is too much for your abdominal muscles, a light girdle might be advised.)

Care of the abdomen.

During pregnancy, in order to accommodate the increasing size of the baby, the fibrous band (the linea alba) formed between the two rectus muscles that run vertically on either side of the centre line of the abdomen, stretches an average of

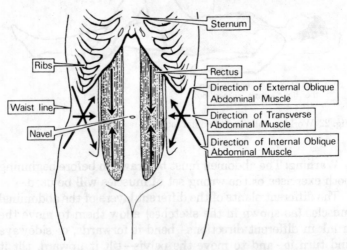

Fig. 23 Direction of abdominal muscle fibres forming a perfect natural corset.

four inches. It cannot return to its former state and size because it is not composed of elastic fibres. It can therefore be the cause of the protrusion of abdominal organs after childbirth if the mother does not know how to keep her abdominal muscles in good condition and to tone up her recti muscles so that they can meet in mid line and obliterate the gap. This must be dealt with after baby's birth by simple exercises. (Fig. 23.)

The skin as well as the muscles of the abdomen stretches during pregnancy and can be kept comfortable by massage and oiling, and also by abdominal exercise. Sit down and stoop slightly forward to relax the abdominal muscles, then, using some oil on the hands as a lubricant (olive or castor), pick up as much of the skin covering the abdomen as possible, bit by bit, and pass it from one hand to the other. This may help to render the skin more elastic. It is valuable chiefly in reducing the irritation which is sometimes felt in the last few weeks as a result of the stretching of the skin.

Exercise 12: muscle control

Lie on the floor or on a bed. Contract all muscles of one arm or one leg and then fully relax, while the rest of the body is completely slack.

Progress by contracting the muscles of both arms while both legs are relaxed and then slacken completely. Change by contracting the legs.

Contract all muscles on one side of the body and keep the other side slack.

Lying on the back with knees bent and feet flat. (1) Pull your abdominal muscles in and let both closed knees fall towards the side of the bed, use your hands to help to sit up, drop the lower legs over the edge of the bed and stand up. Use this procedure every time you change from the lying position to the standing position and so avoid stretching the abdominal muscles.

(2) Slowly relax each knee until both knees touch the floor on their own side. The muscles on the inside of both thighs and the pelvic floor muscles must be completely relaxed. Now add a strong abdominal contraction without tightening up any other muscles.

3. LABOUR

Labour is the natural culmination of pregnancy and means just *work*—(not pain as is so frequently thought). It is said to take place in three stages—first, second and third—but throughout a squeezing of the uterus or womb (the hollow muscular organ in which the baby lives for the first nine months of his life) occurs at regular intervals. This squeezing of a muscle is called a 'contraction' and is often misnamed a 'labour pain'. The uterus is not the only hollow organ in the body which expels its contents with effective relaxation as both the rectum and the bladder do this in a comparable manner. Neither of these expulsive acts is normally accompanied by pain; rather they may be regarded as one of the primitive pleasures, as observation of any normal small child will prove. The reason why this squeezing of the uterus in a normal labour is sometimes painful to many unprepared women is explained on the grounds that through ignorance they are afraid, and this fear tightens the neck of the uterus (the cervix) (Fig. 2) and its lower part, so that the contractions push the baby against a resistance and that hurts. With the pain, fear increases, making the tension (tightness) greater and bringing *more* pain still, and so a vicious circle of pain, fear, and tension is established. However, if a woman learns about labour and realises that the uterine contractions can, in a peaceful and happy atmosphere, actually open the

26

cervix more quickly, she will find that she usually does not experience any strong sensation she is not prepared to meet. If the discomfort becomes unacceptable she should not hesitate to ask for help. This is very often given in the form of inhalation analgesia, which does not harm the baby but often benefits it. The first stage of labour lasts until the cervix is wide open, and then the mother must get to work and start pushing her baby out. This pushing opens out the birth canal (vagina and vulva) and stretches the skin and muscles between the vulva and the anus (perineum). This pushing and the contractions of the uterus eventually push the baby out through the open door of the cervix. This terminates the second stage and the baby is born. The third stage consists (a) of the expulsion of the afterbirth (the placenta), the sponge-like organ attached to the wall of the uterus through which the baby has drawn its food from the mother's blood, (b) of the bag in which the baby has lived within the uterus, and (c) of the cord which has been attached to the placenta at one end and to the baby's navel at the other and through which the nourishment has passed. The placenta is very often immediately removed by the attendant after the baby is born.

Procedure when labour starts

First, it is important to know that the *sensation* may be either a *backache* or abdominal discomfort. It is surprising how many women refuse to believe they are in labour because that is all they feel. It is difficult to give any hard and fast rule about the way labour begins. The main variations in the order of their most frequent occurence are:

A. A 'show'—a menstrual period appears to be starting, often following a call to empty the bowels at a rather unusual time. This may come some days before labour starts properly, or it may come *after B*.

B. A backache sensation as if a period were about to begin, which comes and goes, usually at regular intervals. This will

27

certainly come sooner or later, and may follow the show at once. It is accompanied by a hardening of the uterus which can be felt by putting the hands on the abdominal wall.

C. Rupture of the membranes (the bag in which the baby lives in the uterus) with a gush or trickle of fluid that is not urine. This occurs in only a small percentage of women, as usually the membranes rupture later in labour.

The mother should report at once any of these symptoms to her hospital, doctor or midwife who will give further instructions. These she should follow implicitly and she should promptly report any change that occurs.

Stage I

When labour is established the uterine contractions will come at *intervals,* usually at quite long ones in the beginning, varying from an hour or more to ten minutes or less. Each lasts a few seconds (the average is said to be thirty early in the first stage) and then passes away completely.

Most women prefer to continue their daily routine for a while and this is an excellent decision if the doctor agrees. Usually it is wise to start relaxation about the time when the contractions come at ten- to five-minute intervals, when they will be stronger and be lasting for a longer time (probably up to a minute).

The mother should choose whichever position she prefers and relax instantly and completely each time a contraction begins, not forgetting to breathe using the abdominal wall as described in Exercise 1 (*a*). These contractions are frequently referred to as 'pains' by doctors and midwives, but, as has been said, feel like a dull backache, but *with effective relaxation as labour advances they do not become any sensation the mother is not prepared to experience.* They do, however, increase in strength and length and the intervals between them decrease until the cervix is fully open (dilated).

During the later part of Stage I the mother will find that breathing using the abdominal wall during a contraction

28

becomes almost impossible and is exhausting. She should now adopt a different procedure. During contraction: With rising contraction take a deep breath and immediately release air without abdominal effort. During continuing contraction upper chest breathing—exercise 1 (c)—should be carried out to the height of the contraction. When the contraction subsides revert to deeper abdominal breathing, when the contraction has completely passed away, make a conscious expiratory effort (not forced) and then continue to breathe fully and quietly.

Should the sensations become very strong during the later part of Stage I, the mother should not hesitate to ask for help or accept it when offered by her attendant.

Stage II

After the cervix is dilated the baby must usually be expelled by an active effort on the part of the mother. She will usually be asked to lie on her back, raised on a back support, or with the father's support, the head well bent forward and with her knees bent exactly to the same degree as in the squatting exercise (Exercise 10) she will put her arms round her thighs or knees, or hold her feet, depending upon her own choice. Breathing as described in Exercise 10 (g) is now started, taking in the breath and holding it and then using the 'bearing down' movement. This is similar to the action of emptying the bowels but should be felt in the vagina. This 'pushing' must be forward and not towards the back passage. The 'pushing' can be used only as long as the contraction lasts and then the mother must relax on her back, but this time probably with legs straight and spread apart and arms as in Exercise 4 (Fig. 7). This is all repeated, breathing as in Exercise (g) or (f) as directed by the attendant, with each contraction, until the baby is born.

It will be noticed that holding the breath and 'bearing down' has been recommended as a practice in pregnancy during the natural daily action which takes place in a similar way, that is the emptying of the bowels (Chapter 1). Foot-stools or a bench of suitable height was recommended to be placed in front of the lavatory seat and the feet put on this with the body slightly stooped over and the head drooped (the squatting position of Exercise V) and the bowels were then to be emptied by taking a breath and holding it while bearing down and relaxing the pelvic floor muscles. A daily practice of this therefore became a daily practice of the second stage of labour without strain.

Stage III

The mother has no further part to play but to enjoy the fruits of her labour, and the more fully she is able to do this the more satisfactorily the afterbirth will probably come away. The cord will be cut and then the baby wrapped and given to her to hold at once if she has asked that this may be so.

Post-script: If the doctor decides to induce labour artificially, the timing of the three stages of labour will be altered. The mother's participation, however, in using breathing exercises and muscle control as previously described does not funda-mentally change. She should still follow the instructions of her attendant and actively take part in the birth of her baby.

Combined mental and physical events

The essential exercises practised during pregnancy having now been fitted into labour it is important next to lay the mental (or emotional) foundations. The success of labour depends upon the mother's understanding of her reactions and feelings and upon her realising that labour calls for con-trol, skill, effort and patience, and like other physical feats is a character-building undertaking. She will need all the same attributes to be a successful mother to her family later.

Stage I

Just as a pregnant woman changes and tends to grow healthier, happier, and better looking, so during labour a woman changes and should know that this will be so. It is not uncommon that near the expected date, even for some weeks before, a feeling of impatience and frustration grows. Possibly it is nature's method of increasing the desire for the child's birth. As labour starts this gives way to excitement and exhilaration, a 'wanting to tell everyone'. This lasts until the cervix is about half dilated, the mother gradually becoming more serious and realising that her work has now inevitably to be done. It is the *inevitableness* that at this stage brings some element of doubt and even fear into almost all women's minds. What they have heard from friends and relations, what they have read, all tend to rise to the surface. This is one time when their preparation serves them well. They have learned what they will have to do and because of their reading and practice, feel confident they can do it well. They have noticed uterine contractions probably for some weeks, though without the sensation in the back, and *now* realise that their accompaniment is a faint ache in the lower back, so slight that with happy occupation and mental ease it may be ignored for hours and even throughout labour. If it grows in intensity, it can be relieved by firm pressure or rubbing, by the husband or another attendant, over the sacral region (lower back just above the buttocks). Labour sensations are generally all in the back, the rectum and the vaginal outlet. (A few women have the sensation in the abdomen.) A well-prepared mother, *with a suitable person in attendance when she needs it* to exhort her to further effort and to encourage her or to correct any faults that occur, will continue with her relaxation and muscle control and gradually become aware of the onset of the second stage. Some or all of the following changes will be present:

Transition stage (between the first and second stages)

(1) The mother will experience inability to make the abdominal wall move by breathing during a contraction, thus making complete relaxation with a contraction no longer possible in the old way—breathing should now be done as in Exercise 1 (c).

(2) The contractions will have narrowed down to about two- or three-minute intervals and it will be noticed that there has been no more shortening of the interval for some time.

(3) There will be a growing awareness of a lump in the rectum as of a very large stool to be passed. It is the pressure of the baby's head against the rectum, through the wall of the vagina (Fig. 2).

(4) A catch in the breath comparable to a 'belch' appears at intervals. It is the first attempt of the diaphragm to establish the expulsive efforts.

(5) This action of the diaphragm may produce a desire to vomit and the mother will have learned that she can close her mouth and swallow and press downward slightly to check the desire. Vomiting may occur but is of no significance and many women vomit once or twice at this stage.

(6) Violent shaking, as if excited. Enough to make the teeth chatter in some cases. It is just a nervous reaction—nothing to worry about. Holding the breath does sometimes help.

(7) Cramp in the buttocks and thighs, sometimes down the outside of the legs. Stretching the legs between contractions will help.

(8) An involuntary bearing down movement of the abdominal wall—never experienced at any other time and most interesting and entertaining to feel when it is expected and understood. It must *not* be used for bearing down until dilatation is complete, therefore the panting breathing of Exercise 10 or inhalation analgesia must be adopted to prevent the breath being held, and the abdominal wall becoming contracted.

(9) Rupture of the membranes, which may go occasionally

with a distinct 'pop' but does not hurt. Membranes can rupture before labour starts or at *any* time during labour.

(10) Gradually the chest breathing will change in nature and the expiration particularly will include a faint groaning sound, the mother experiencing increasingly the desire—to 'bear down'. This eventually becomes so strong that only the panting breaths of Exercise 10 or inhalation analgesia can prevent it.

A woman in labour should never bear down deliberately until permission is given by her medical attendant or midwife —she should pant to prevent breath-holding and contraction of the abdominal wall.

Stage II

Once her own suspicions are confirmed by the attendant and she is told that her cervix is fully open and she may begin to expel, she will experience a very great change. Whereas her whole being has been concentrating upon breathing and muscle control, possibly in some trepidation, now she will find her mood changes and she becomes completely sure of herself and settles down to concentrate on a job which exists in a world of its own.

Between bearing down efforts amnesia (unawareness of surroundings) is often marked so that the mother will not hear questions or remarks, and she *may* even profess herself 'too tired' to make any more effort as the stage goes on. All the same, each time a uterine contraction occurs the effort to bear down is resumed and the mother realises that she is growing heated and perspiring exactly as if she was doing strenuous work. Gradually she begins to feel the child in the vagina instead of the rectum and the time for which she has been waiting draws near. She knows that soon a very obvious stretching feeling will be experienced which sometimes even amounts to a feeling of splitting open. This must not arouse alarm, as it is not painful when the muscles are well prepared. It should be *appreciated* as it is the prelude to the birth of the

33

head. Round about this stage the mother may be asked to pant softly as in Exercise 10 (*f*), instead of bearing down, so that the baby's head can be born more gently. She must at this point listen very carefully for instructions and put them into action at once.

As the head is born she will feel her first sensation of release and can if she wishes watch the body come. Within a minute she may see the baby completely born, and here she has such a rush of feelings—physical and mental, joy and release and elation—that one cannot attempt to describe it to her. She will watch the baby's first movements, listen to its first cry, and as soon as the cord is cut she will want to hold it in her arms bundled up in its blanket, velvet soft and warm in all its perfection.

Stage III

The mother's work is now over and the midwife delivers the placenta. A third feeling of relief will be experienced, a physical relief of quite surprising magnitude, and the delight in finding the abdomen flat once more has to be experienced to be believed. Here the mother may be interested in seeing the placenta, a cord and membranes, and should ask them to be shown if she so desires.

When all this is over she will feel extremely fit and well and probably ravenously hungry and thirsty. She will respond to all suggestions happily and state herself ready to get up at once, even though she knows this will not be allowed. She will want her baby near her, and be ready to feed it as soon as it is washed and dressed and comfortable, or even before.

The husband

What of the newly made father, who has prepared himself for the event of the birth of the child he has helped to create? An increasing number of parents are beginning to share in natural childbirth, and where both of you are prepared and wish it, you should make enquiries if this is possible for you. There is no doubt that it perfects the experience for both. Even to be together for *part* of the time, especially at the end of the first stage, which is acknowledged to be the most difficult part of labour and often gives the mother a sense of great loneliness, brings great benefit and comfort.

This little book can, however, close on no better note than in the words of a young father who had been helping his wife throughout labour: 'If I live to be a hundred I shall never see anything more wonderful'.